ALCOHOL... So, You Want the TRUTH?

with CHERYL'S STORY

Joseph G. Apple

February, 2019

"No safe level of alcohol," Lancet editor, Richard Horton.[1]

"...safest level of drinking is none" Emmanuela Gakidou, professor of Health Metrics and Evaluation, University of Washington.[2]

"...champagne, wine, beer... good for you? ...none are correct." Max Griswold, senior researcher, University of Washington School of Medicine.[3]

I'm still waiting for people to get it.

Alcohol is nothing more than a mind-altering, feel-good, poisonous drug. When used as an antiseptic, it kills germs. When used as a beverage, it kills people.

Beverage alcohol is toxic to the human body. The only reason it does not kill us with the first drink is because our bodies possess enzymes to detoxify it. That alone defines ethyl alcohol as toxic to the human body.

The enzymes alcohol dehydrogenase, hydrogenase, catalase and cytochrome p450 break ethyl alcohol down to acetaldehyde, which travels to the liver to be oxidized and eliminated from the body.

The acetaldehyde molecule is very harmful to living tissue and wreaks its own havoc as it courses through the body before being flushed out...think "cirrhosis of the liver."[4] Alcohol is also implicated in cancers of the mouth, throat, larynx, esophagus, pancreas and stomach.

Alcohol weakens the *brakes* on everything.

Chapter 6 of the Montana Driver Manual reports that, "Alcohol reduces all of the important skills needed to drive safely and will affect your brain within one minute of consumption." It goes on to say:

"Alcohol affects the areas that control judgment and skill...that you will not know when to stop drinking until it is too late."[5]

Alcohol slows your reactions, reduces your ability to see clearly and makes you less alert. The more you drink...the dumber you are.

The driver manual also states that, "Microbrews and craft beers often contain more alcohol than a 12-ounce commercial beer and are often the same as having several drinks."

The driver manual continues by saying, "Fifty per cent of all fatal traffic accidents in Montana are alcohol-related, and 23,000 deaths nationwide are caused each year by alcohol."[5]

You see the red traffic-light and truly intend to stop in time...but surprise! ...you end up in the middle of the intersection.

According to a 2017 study conducted by Montana Attorney General, Tim Fox, "...alcohol was involved in half of all suicides in the year 2013." His study continues to report, "...alcohol and drugs cost the state $1.4 million with 20,000 hospital ER visits yearly."

The study shows that statistically, "...one of every ten Montanans is dependent on alcohol or drugs." Also, "...61% of Montana high school students who drink, binge-drink."

Mr. Fox's report also states:

"...37.7 of 100,000 Montana deaths were as a result of alcohol consumption...**the highest rate in the nation.**" Additionally, "...24% of rapes in Montana had an alcohol component in 2015," which he felt was actually underreported.

Theft, burglary and criminal endangerment offenses carry a high level of alcohol involvement with a 63% increase since 2009.[6]

A Montana sheriff survey reports Montana's jail population to be 89-95% full, which is the highest occupancy rate in the nation. In the years 2012-2016, 40% of all felony convictions carried a drugs or alcohol component.

Also, 58% of all convictions in that time period were either deferred or suspended. Forty-two per cent of the guilty parties were sentenced to the Department of Corrections or prison.

According to the survey, the average cost of a prison stay is $80,798 for males and $57,780 for females.

The most frequent offenses are for DUI, drug use and drug distribution. Bill Hooks, former Montana Public Defender chief advises:

"We need to do a lot more to prevent them from ever coming into the system."[7]

As a hospital volunteer in the emergency room of Kalispell Regional Hospital, I have personally sat with numb family members as they waited to hear the results concerning loved ones after an alcohol-related event.

One tragic day, a teen son, father and uncle were transported to the ER after a successful youth deer hunt. The boy had bagged a deer, which was in the bed of the truck as they headed home.

The driver had consumed one or more alcoholic drinks and had misjudged a curve in the road. The truck rolled several times, ejecting all 3 members. One man died quickly while the other man clung to life for another 6 days before being removed from life-support. The 13-yr-old boy suffered several broken bones and internal injuries, but survived.

This event was reported in Kalispell's <u>Daily Inter Lake</u> newspaper on September 8, 2015, but they did not have the final news concerning the event. They reported that alcohol was indeed involved as a contributing factor in the crash.

I sat with the shocked wife in the hospital's waiting room as we talked about which vegetables to soon plant in our gardens...while her husband lay dead in back...but she did not know just yet.

I would expect that our mayor and city council members would be eager to address the alcohol problem in Kalispell. But sadly, that does not seem to be the case.

New alcohol licenses are granted each year, reaping a huge financial windfall. In the years

2017 and 2018, **$2,278,000** was reported from alcohol permits granted.

The list from city records is as follows:

3-13-17	Blue Samurai	$150,000
5-25-17	Casa Mexico	$800,000
5-19-17	Staggering Ox	$30,000
2-1-17	Magic Diamond Casino	$250,000
1-30-17	Montana Lil's Casino	$350,000
4-11-18	Scottibelli's	$50,000
5-31-18	Kobe Steakhouse & Sushi	$102,000
10-1-18	Players Club Casino	$500,000
12-19-18	Urban Bricks Pizza	$46,000[8]

Some of the licenses may have been transactions between license owners, but still, alcohol permits are very profitable for *someone*.

Our Kalispell, Montana newspaper, the <u>Daily</u> <u>Inter Lake</u>, takes part in promoting alcohol events. On January 13, 2019, I read the heading:

"Kalispell Brewfest Celebrates Craft Beers."

"...outdoor events for the whole family."

"...a kids' dash-for-cash."

"...children under 12 free."

"...hosted by Valley Bank."

"...proceeds go to Kalispell Downtown Association and Flathead Community Foundation."

And again, on February 3, 2019, the <u>Daily Inter Lake</u> promotes alcohol advertising by devoting a full half-page to talk about a bill in favor of expanding brewery serving hours in Whitefish, Montana.

One possible bright note comes from Joe Unterreiner, Director of Kalispell Chamber of Commerce, who stated in the <u>Daily Inter Lake</u> on January 16, 2019 that he supports, "common-sense changes to liquor laws." It will be interesting to see what he means by, "common sense."

So much money is made from alcohol sales that no one wants to look at the ugly consequences. City leaders want the increased profits from alcohol taxes while pretending the problem belongs to someone else.

The ugly truth is that our citizens are dying daily from the effects of alcohol consumption. It is not *alcohol abuse,* but alcohol *consumption.*

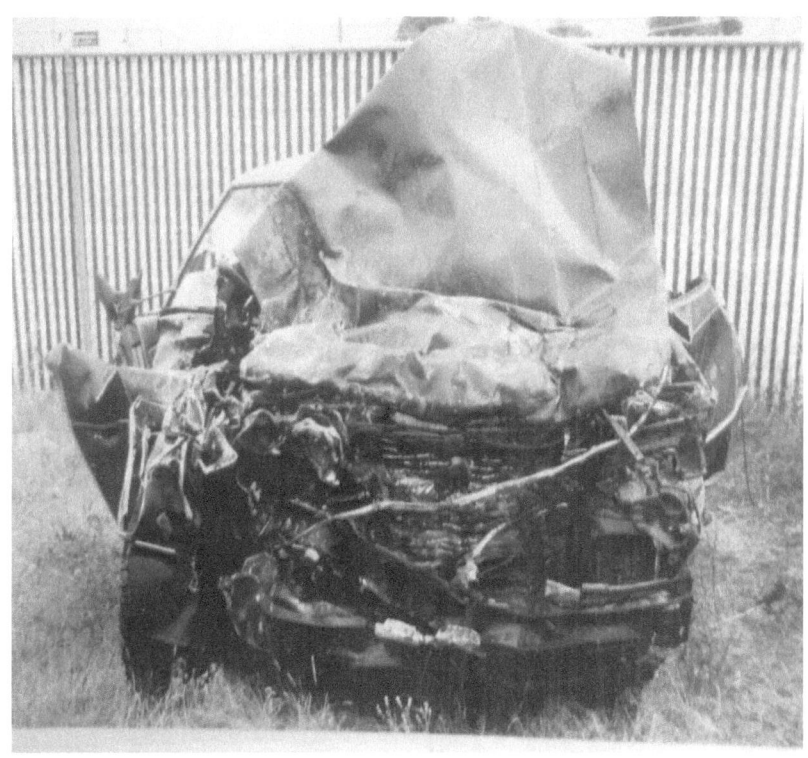

My friend, Cheryl Ward was riding in the car above. I will get to that later.

Binge-drinking is reported to be a big problem among high school and college students. The question is sometimes asked:

"Just how much alcohol does it take to kill a person?"

Mike Pearl reports on that question for the publication, Vice. He states that the answer depends on several factors, the most important being a person's weight or body-size.

In his reporting, he determines the "magic" blood alcohol concentration level to be around the 0.34% level. He mentions that anywhere between the 0.30% and 0.40% mark will *get you there*.

 "People have been known to die at those levels," Pearl says.

To state the matter in more practical terms, Pearl says it would take about 14 shots of whiskey to get an average-size person such as himself to that 0.34% mark...between stupor and death.[31]

George Koob, director of the National Institute on Alcohol Abuse and Alcoholism at the National Institutes of Health also comments on the amount of alcohol required to cause death...

"...a whole bottle of Scotch...17 shots...or less with 101-Wild Turkey."

Koob informs us that, "Drinking alcohol causes a release of dopamine and other chemicals that make the drinker 'feel nice.' But that feeling stops after a while and the experience starts to become grueling around the 0.08% BAC mark...where you are too drunk to drive."

He goes on to say, "The average person then starts thinking maybe drinking a little more alcohol will make it fun again?...and that's the point where you're liable to black out...somewhere around a BAC of 0.20%.

The seriously drunk individual often dies from drowning in their own vomit because the "gag reflex" no longer works properly. If you have a choice about it, you might want to avoid this one.

For a good rule-of thumb, Koob estimates the average person could easily kill themselves by drinking, "...fifteen standard drinks [of hard liquor] in two hours." But he advises that no one try it.[32]

According to the people at Alcohol.org, they agree that consuming about one quart of hard liquor all at once will kill the average person.[33]

I am curious if alcohol were to be introduced to the public today, in 2019, if the Food and Drug Administration would even allow it. The window between intoxication and death looks to be very narrow.

Six or seven gulps of 101-Wild Turkey seem to be enough to kill a guy.

I was working a shift in the ER of a California hospital on a Saturday night when a comatose male wearing a tuxedo was wheeled in. He had been brought in from a wedding celebration. His friends said the guy had "guzzled" a large amount of gin, "...all at once."

The male was intubated and placed on a ventilator. He was unconscious during the remainder of my shift. A couple of the male nurses took a photo of the man using his own phone and placed the photo on his phone's screen-saver. They wanted him to know exactly what he looked like with all the medical equipment hooked to his body, keeping him alive.

Sarah M. Hartz, assistant professor of psychiatry at Washington University in Saint Louis shares the results after an alcohol study involving 400,000 people, ages 18-85. The international team, which included hundreds of researchers, examined data from more than 1,000 studies. It is the largest compilation of alcohol data so far.

The results from the study show that...

"Drinking a daily glass of wine for health reasons may not be so healthy after all."

The study showed how drinking one-to-two drinks, four times per week increases the risk of death across all age groups by 20%.

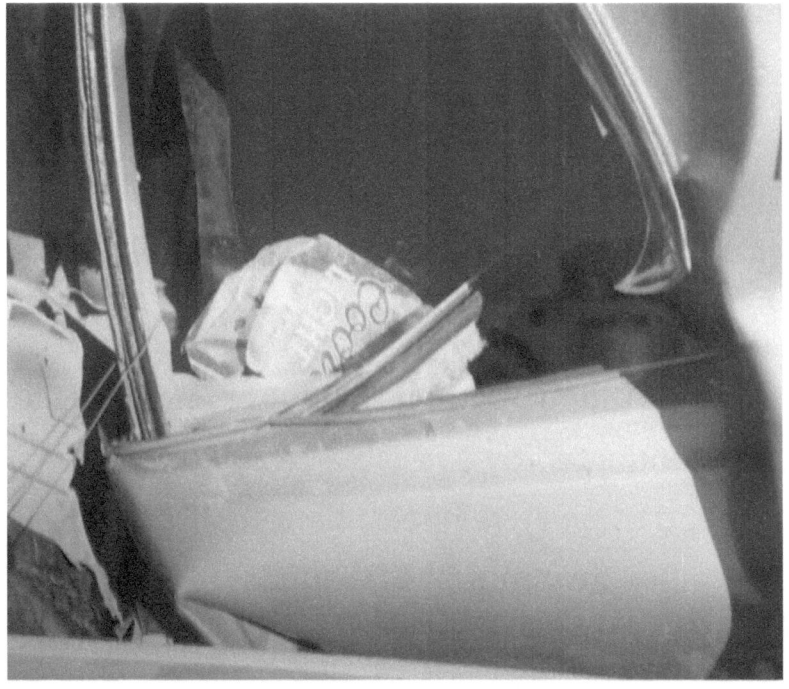

Photo above: The car that killed Vernon Ward, Cheryl Ward's husband.

She went on to say, "…now we know that even the lightest daily drinkers have an increased mortality risk."[30]

I have read of many doctors who said it was good, or healthy to daily drink a glass of wine. But there is no medical proof to support such a claim. Physicians are not supposed to advise behaviors that have not been proven to be medically sound and true.

I have not found even one double-blind medical study conducted by a reliable research group that reports positive health benefits from consuming any amount of alcohol. It does not seem to exist.

Why do physicians advise such a thing? I wonder if physicians are rewarded by alcohol providers in any way. Or, are they just trying to keep their drinking-patients happy in an effort to maintain a *positive cash-flow*?

I confronted the pastor of my local church about his accepting "drinkers" into church membership. In my faith, we do not condone the usage of tobacco products or the consumption of beverage alcohol.

He told me he wanted to keep the people, "happy." I hope he wasn't rebelling against the rules in order to keep the church afloat. In the end, these things are usually about money.

The National Institute on Alcohol Abuse and Alcoholism (NIAAA) says an estimated 88,000 people (62,000 men, 26,000 women) die each year from alcohol-related causes and is the 3rd leading cause of preventable deaths.[9]

Public records show that alcohol companies spend close to $2 billion yearly on advertising in the Unites States alone. From 2001-2007, they aired more than 2 million TV ads and published more than 20,000 magazine ads.[10]

According to Budweiser chief executive officer, Joao Castro Neves, after losing ground to craft beers, Budweiser plans to spend **$2 billion** themselves to promote their drinks through the year 2020.[11]

Montana is big on "craft beers," ranking 3rd in the nation per capita, according to a Sept. 15, 2014 article in the Flathead Beacon.

Dartmouth University Pediatrician, James D. Sargent says more than 80% of movies depict alcohol usage. He did not offer proof, but assumes the alcohol companies are paying for it.

As an example, he spoke of the 2003 "good-natured family comedy," Elf, and how alcohol was introduced as Will Ferrell, playing Elf, poured whiskey into his coffee, which started an office party. [12] As a follow-up, there is also an Elf "drinking game," which the providers of the game suggest be played with *hard liquor*.

Karoline Knorr, in "Parenting, Media and Everything in Between," from <u>Common Sense Media</u> stated, "...according to a 2006 study, each additional dollar spent on ads raises the number of drinks youths consume by 3%."

She added, **"Kids who start drinking before the age of 15 are 4 times more likely to become alcoholics than those who begin after the age of 21."[13]**

It should come as no surprise that alcohol companies are targeting our children.

While allowable on cable, broadcast television rules do not allow actual consumption of alcoholic beverages to take place in alcohol commercials. But alcohol providers work around that rule by getting alcohol incorporated into the programs themselves.

Lance Strate, Professor of Communication and Media Studies at Fordham University, notes that, "If the advertisers can't show how cool drinking is, the programs can."

He speaks of how TV programs such as, <u>How I Met Your Mother,</u> and <u>Cougar Town,</u> are nothing but blatant advertisements for alcohol.[14]

We know that tobacco companies got away with this for many years as they paid actors to "light up" in movie scenes. It seems that alcohol companies are now getting away with it.

Daily TV programs such as, <u>The Today Show,</u> have full glasses of wine prominently displayed in front of the hosts, as though to suggest that this is a normal part of anyone's day.

Alcohol pours freely on the TV show, <u>The Bachelor,</u> as beautiful women sip wine in practically *every-other-scene.*

I just witnessed a 2019 Super Bowl commercial where Budweiser claimed to be using "wind power" to make their brew. Is the "wind power" supposed to make it natural?

Budweiser learned long ago how to play on human emotions by featuring Clydesdale horses and Dalmatian dogs in their beer commercials.

Am I the only one to see through this drivel?...how a little Clydesdale pony wants to grow up and be like his "daddy" and someday help pull the Budweiser wagon?...and does no one else see how this is an emphasis on pushing alcohol onto the kids?...really?

And if beer-drinkers think they are drinking "American beers,"...think again.

Budweiser, Michelob and Busch are all owned by "InBev," a conglomerate that owns over 250 breweries based in **Belgium and Brazil.**[34]

Miller Beer is owned by "SABMiller," a brewery based in **South Africa.** The "SAB" stands for, South Africa **B**eer.[34]

Pabst has no breweries of their own but contracts their beer out to SABMiller...and you now know where that is located. It makes little difference, but Pabst was recently bought by a **Russian** company that goes by the name of, "Oasis."[35]

Heineken International Beer is produced by a **Dutch** brewing company, so there is nothing American there.

Coors is owned by "Molson Coors Brewing Co.," based in **Canada.** They call themselves a "North American Beer," which is technically true since Canada and the United States are both part of the "North American continent."

Why does this remind me of *quilted toilet paper* that is wrapped more loosely to give me less product with increased profits for the manufacturer?

They don't put it quite like that, but I think you get the idea who gets it in the end.

Budweiser has introduced flavored alcoholic drinks that sound more like fruit drinks and sodas. Now, who is that aimed at?

As a reminder, the purchase of alcoholic drinks is still illegal under the age of 18 in most states. The age limit here in Montana is 21.

Why should any of this matter?

In the year 1995, according to the Substance Abuse and Mental Health Services Administration, the total cost to The United States was $166.5 **billion** per year in lost wages and productivity.[10]

In 2010, The Center for Disease Control estimated the total cost to the United States for alcohol abuse was $249 **billion**[29] annually, which amounts to an increase of $5.5 **billion** per year over those 15 years.

If that increase has continued at the same pace, the total alcohol burden to the U.S. economy in the year 2019 should be approximately $298.5 **billion** per year, which is well over **one-quarter trillion dollars.**

Montana's lawmakers do not seem to be concerned about the problem. Some lawmakers are even casino and tavern owners themselves. Montana congressman, Ed Buttrey, admits that he holds a "small beverage license" and owns several liquor and casino establishments, as reported in the <u>Montana Standard</u>.[15]

I must ask the question...

Isn't this like a fox with a bed in the hen house?

All states in the Union were graded in a 2017 study by wallethub.com. The states were ranked concerning DUI penalties and prevention.

Of all 50 states, Montana was ranked towards the bottom at number "40" overall. Montana was number "21" in penalties, and number "47" in prevention.

Arizona was the strictest with the ranking of "1" in penalties, and "2" in prevention.[16]

In Arizona, the first DUI results in the automobile being impounded. The offender is hit with 10 days in jail with a fine of $750. The second DUI results in 90 days spent in jail and a fine of $1,750. The offender's driver's license is also suspended for 90 days with the first DUI.

In Arizona, a mandatory ignition breathalyzer/interlock device must be installed after the first DUI at a cost to the driver of approximately $1,000. The interlock device must remain in place for one full year.[17]

It is easy to see how driving under the influence of alcohol has been drastically reduced in the state of Arizona due to their severe penalties.

In Montana, anyone convicted of a DUI loses their driver's license for at least 90 days.[18] But that charge does not stop offenders from driving. One of the most frequent court charges I see posted in the newspaper is, "driving while suspended."

Montana is the worst of all the states in the union concerning highway deaths attributed to alcohol, with the most DUI fatalities per miles driven.[19]

According to a 2010 study by the University of Montana, it was announced that DUI offenders in Montana reported driving under the influence of alcohol **369 times** for each DUI conviction he or she received. This total was also thought to be under-reported.[20]

In Montana, the minimum jail-time for the first DUI is one day. A second DUI brings a jail-stay of 7 days, but may be lowered at a judge's discretion. I have noticed that the usual time spent in jail is indeed, *one day.* The recommended minimum fine for the first DUI is $600-$1,000, left to the judge's discretion.[21] In January, 2019, I currently see fines of $850.

Montana allows 4 DUIs before it becomes a felony.[22] That means the offender may drive an automobile approximately **1,476 times** while under the influence of alcohol before being classified as a felon.

The University of Montana document continued by stating, "...the average DUI conviction in

Montana occurred when the offender's blood alcohol concentration level (BAC) was 0.16%, which is twice the legal limit of 0.08%."[23]

Utah recently lowered their maximum blood alcohol concentration level from 0.08% to 0.05% for intoxicated motorists. The event would automatically become a felony if a death was involved. Utah legislators are urging all states to adopt the 0.05% BAC standard.[24]

Montana's maximum blood alcohol concentration level is 0.08 per cent. A BAC level of 0.08% or higher warrants a driving-under-the-influence (DUI) charge.[25]

On a more personal note, my friend Cheryl Ward, a swimming coach at Kalispell's health center, The Summit, shares her story involving a drunk motorist.[26]

Cheryl and Her husband, Vernon (Vern), were driving to Missoula, Montana, 125 miles south of Kalispell, on the morning of August 4, 1990 where Cheryl was to participate in a triathlon sporting event (swim-bike-run). In 1990, Cheryl was 46 and Vernon was 51.

They opted to make the drive that morning rather than the previous evening in hopes of avoiding any possible intoxicated motorists on the road. Cheryl says:

"We wanted to be back in Kalispell before the drunks were on the road. Also, there was a wedding at our church and we hoped to be back in time to attend."

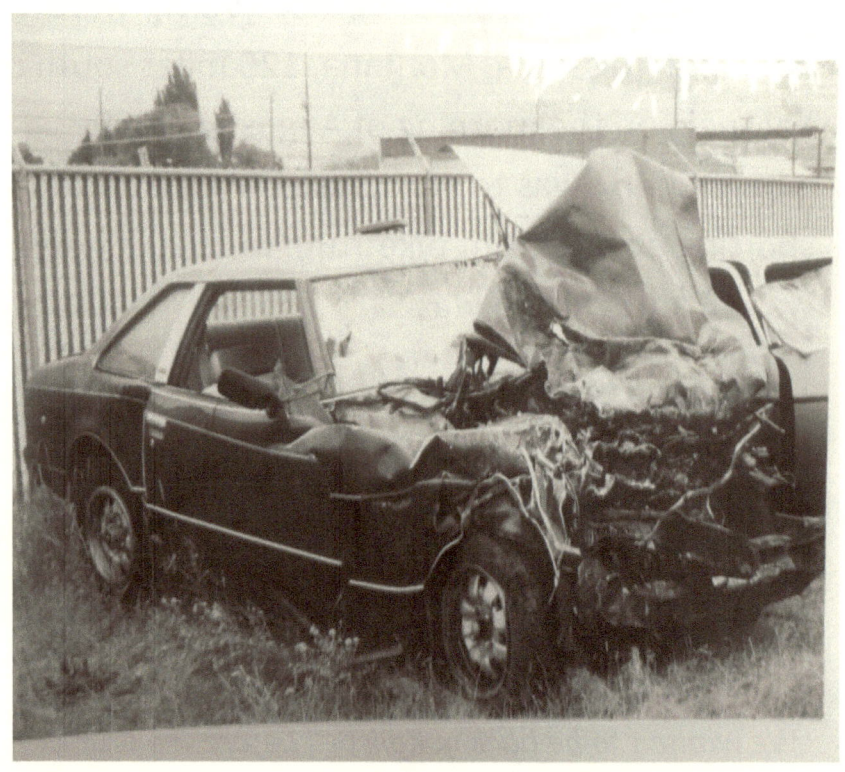

Cheryl recalls that as Vern drove on a section of Highway 93 South known as, Evaro Hill, a "20s woman with a passenger" approached them from the opposite direction...swerved into their lane, and crashed into their car, "head-on."

Cheryl recalls that the accident took place around 8:00 a.m. that morning.

"Vern always drove near the speed limit. They said the other driver was going about 90 mph. We were hit head-on and Vern and the other driver were killed."

Cheryl recalls that the drunk woman was driving on a **suspended license** with **no insurance.**

Both Cheryl's husband, Vernon, and the female driver in the other automobile were killed instantly. Vernon had planned on watching their 3-yr-old granddaughter, Caroline, that morning while Cheryl, her daughter Susan, and son-in-law Gary participated in the triathlon.

Cheryl sustained multiple, severe injuries:

...broken jaw, broken and missing teeth, broken right arm, broken left femur, crushed pelvis, 2 broken hips, crushed left foot and both ankles severely broken.

"My memories at the accident site are spotty. I don't remember the impact. I was dozing and thinking about biking when we were hit".

Both Cheryl and Vernon were wearing their seatbelts.

"I don't remember seeing anything. I do remember hearing a voice...an angel, I thought. A vacationing family stopped to help. The lady stayed by me and gave me comfort with her words. I know she made the difference. I think she kept me alive with her voice."

Cheryl did not know where she was or what had happened to her. All she knew was that she wanted to get away from where she was and away from the "excruciating, indescribable pain."

"I do remember hearing a helicopter and hoping that it was not for me because of the cost. I was taken to St. Pat's by ambulance after being extricated from the car with the Jaws of Life."

The helicopter actually was not for Cheryl, but for the injured passenger in the other car who was asleep in the back seat area. Cheryl's severe fractures mandated that she be transported by ambulance since that would be less bumpy.

"I thought I was moaning...maybe from the pain. A friend of mine who came upon the scene told me she heard 'God-awful screaming' coming from the car."

At the triathlon, Cheryl's daughter, Susan, knew something was wrong when her mom and dad did not show. Ironically, Cheryl's name was drawn for the top raffle prize at the event, but she had to be physically present in order to claim it. **The drunk driver robbed her of that too.**

Cheryl was rushed to St. Patrick's Hospital in Missoula where she underwent emergency surgery. She was operated on by orthopedic surgeon, Dr. Woolley, an experienced bone surgeon and pelvis expert who specialized in this type of surgery.

Cheryl recalls her first words to Dr. Woolley after waking from surgery:

"...I asked him when I could run again? I don't know what he said, but I heard, 'six weeks.' What no one told me was that there was a question about whether I would ever walk again."

Doctor Woolley informed her that she looked more like, "road kill!"

He painstakingly put her shattered pelvis back together and inserted a metal rod through her femur. The broken arm was splinted and wrapped. It was to be dealt with later. Future surgeries were planned for her feet and ankles. Cheryl was then confined to a bed for 3 months with strict orders to remain "flat" while her pelvis healed. Her jaw had been wired shut with future jaw surgeries planned.

Cheryl remembers a nurse who caused additional harm:

"I was hurting badly and asked the nurse to move me to get some weight off of one side. She leaned close to me and told me I should take responsibility for my pain. I pulled on the bars of the bed to help myself and pulled apart the bone in my arm. I didn't realize I shouldn't use that hand and arm."

Doctor Woolley operated on that broken arm after all as he added yet more metal and screws to Cheryl's body.

"I then had two metal pins sticking out of my wrist. The rod is still inside and easy to feel. I still think about the nurse who should have done her job and helped me."

A special "air bed" was brought in at an additional cost of $100 per day. Cheryl was in terrible pain, even with the IV morphine drip.

Cheryl was told some flowers had arrived for her.

"I'm not sure which day it was...but I received a large, beautiful bouquet of flowers and note from the lady who comforted me at the accident scene. She called me too. Before that, I thought I imagined the voice."

Doctor Woolley put Cheryl back together with lots of stainless steel and wire. Cheryl comments on all the steel in her body:

"My jaw has metal, and my jaw was wired shut for a while. My pelvis has metal on each side. Looking at an X-ray of my pelvis makes me think I have a metal praying mantis on each side. My left femur had a metal rod and screws. It hurt so badly I later asked him to remove it, which he did. But the pain did not go away, much to my disappointment."

Cheryl's dietician was giving Cheryl a hard time because she thought Cheryl was purposely not eating. Cheryl's weight had dropped from one hundred pounds to seventy-five pounds.

"Extra butter and cream were added to my food which was pureed because of my teeth and wires. Everything I tried was horrible and had almost no taste. I really was trying to eat. They fed me a can of 'Ensure', which I threw up. I still can't look at another can of 'Ensure!' They later inserted tubes down my throat which also really hurt. "

Cheryl later learned that morphine kills a person's appetite.

Cheryl was able to be dismissed from the hospital after a stay of 2 ½ weeks. But since she had to remain "flat," she would need to be transported back home to Kalispell from Missoula by ambulance.

Her insurance provider only allowed that service if it was an "emergency," and balked at funding the necessary transport. Cheryl's aunt and uncle came to her rescue. The passenger seat-back in their car would fold down, allowing Cheryl to be placed in a prone position for the trip back to Kalispell.

With her husband now deceased, Cheryl had to rely on family and friends for her care.

*"My family had rented a hospital bed and reclining wheel-chair for me. Uncle Bill and Gary carefully lifted me out of the car and carried me into the house and bed. I was happy to be home. **But Vern's loss was real at home.** The loss did not seem as real in the hospital."*

Since Cheryl had lost so much weight, her friends did all they could to help get her back to her old self.

Cheryl's sister, Sandy, flew to Kalispell from Georgia to do whatever she could do to help her sis in distress.

"Sandy was a very good nurse, taking excellent care of me....she also took care of our dog and cat."

Other friends pitched in to help Cheryl wherever they could.

"Friends came to my rescue. A good friend from Libby said she would spend a couple of weeks with me after my family left. My youngest son's ex-girlfriend moved in so that she could help."

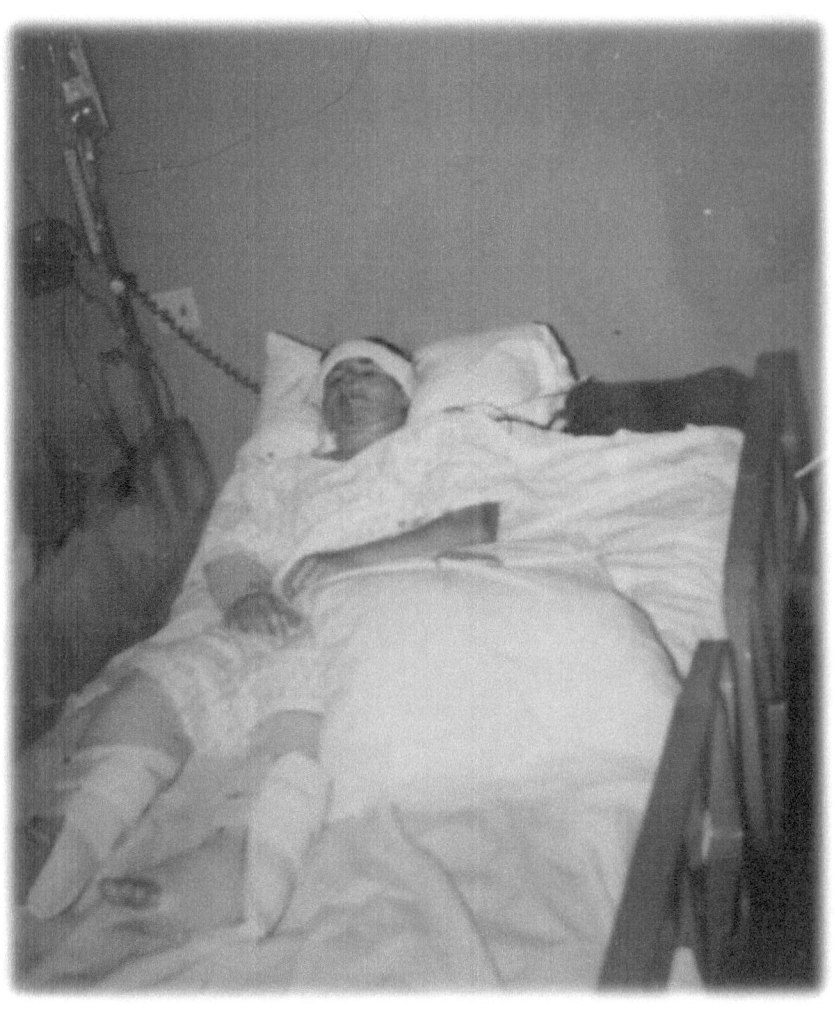

Cheryl's family did all they could, but had their own lives and responsibilities and could not stay long.

Cheryl's husband, Vernon, was now deceased but she was not in any frame of mind to mourn for him. All of her energy had to be focused on surviving.

Cheryl says it was many years after the accident before she finally was able to mourn Vern's passing.

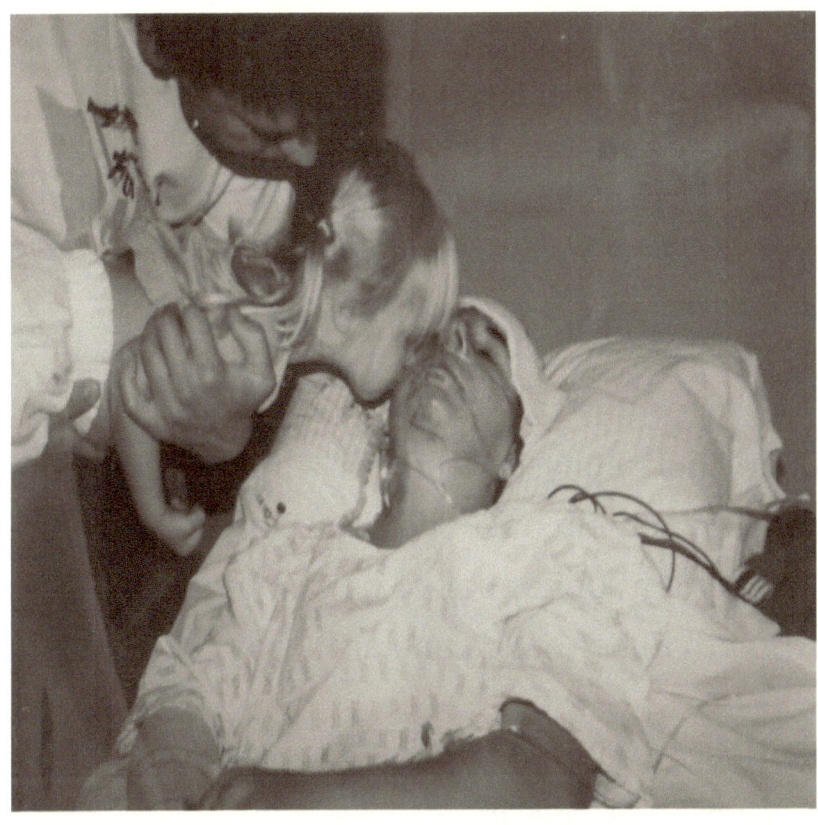

Cheryl's granddaughter, Caroline, does all she can do.

Cheryl knew she had to get better on her own as quickly as possible. She worked hard on rehabilitating her broken body.

"I knew I had to get better before my friends left. I discovered how weak I had gotten in those 2 ½ weeks. A small plate of food was brought to me. I asked for my granddaughter's plastic plate since the other plate was too heavy."

Cheryl had a physical therapist-friend, Kim, who came by to help out. She had Cheryl squeezing putty and a rubber ball to help in regaining strength in her hands and arms.

"I squeezed the ball, first with only my left hand until my right arm healed more, then using both hands. Just doing that made a difference. Kim had me push 'down' on the three-inch foam pad I slept on to get my legs stronger. I was building some strength."

A normal mattress was too painful for Cheryl.

"I had a three-inch-thick foam pad I slept on. I still have pain if I sleep on a mattress without my foam. My body hurt everywhere. I had to sleep with only a thin sheet covering me due to the pain caused by blankets."

Cheryl's friends continued to help her recover after that drunk driver's moment of alcohol-induced insanity.

"I don't remember for sure, but I don't think my hair was washed in the hospital. My friend, Kathy, came to my rescue again...with a tray at the kitchen sink...in my reclining wheel-chair. Boy, it felt so good with clean hair!"

Cheryl's helpers continued to find pieces of glass imbedded in her skin. Cheryl had received numerous cuts and bruises all over her body. Her friend, Kathy, pulled a large piece of overlooked glass from the back of her scalp one day with the words...

"You don't want to know!"

With her jaw wired shut, Cheryl had difficulty getting liquids down, even with a straw.

"With my jaw wired shut, they gave me my pain pills at the hospital by sticking them through the hole in front where one of my teeth used to be."

Once Cheryl was back home in Kalispell, she had follow-up appointments at Kalispell Regional Hospital, but still had to be kept prone due to her shattered pelvis that continued to be very unstable.

Another friend came to her rescue with his pickup truck. It took several people to each grab a corner of the reclining wheelchair and carry her to the truck. She was then gently driven to the hospital...in the bed of a truck.

"My friend, Bob, came over and backed his pickup up to my front porch. I was carried in the reclining wheel chair and placed in the bed of the truck. Men at the hospital carried me inside the hospital where I gave my blood. I thought it was funny that this seemed perfectly normal to them. I'm still surprised."

Cheryl still had a long road of recovery ahead of her. With her husband Vern now deceased and family members returning to their respective homes, her many friends increased their levels of support.

"I am so thankful for the help of my friends; phone company friends, church friends, swim team friends, athlete friends...it seemed the whole community knew of my plight."

Cheryl's friends continued to supply her with food.

"My friend, Dawn, from the phone company lived close by and brought food almost every day. She told me I was looking better every day. I later learned that she told our co-workers I was looking 'terrible' and that they needed to bring more food!"

Cheryl reports that it took her a long time to begin gaining weight.

"Everyone was trying to fatten me up, but it took a while before I weighed 80 pounds."

Cheryl reports that her glasses were destroyed in the crash, which she really missed since she is near-sighted. Cheryl could not recognize her friends when they came to visit in the hospital. Her good friend, Kathy, came to the rescue once again with a unique gift.

"Kathy's head is about the same size as mine and she went to my eye doctor and persuaded him to make glasses with frames that fit 'her head,' but using my prescription. They fit!"

Cheryl also had a brand new bicycle mounted to the back of their vehicle the morning of the crash that had mysteriously disappeared. It was not until several weeks later that she learned the bike had flown a considerable distance in the crash, landing out of sight in a ditch.

"My son, Chris, helped purchase a very expensive racing bike...around $800 I think we paid for it. That was a lot of money for a competition bike just then. He said he would not do that again, thinking he had jinxed me!"

A highway worker found the bike later and took it home, not knowing how it had come to rest in the ditch. He happened to read a news article about Cheryl's misfortune and found a way to reunite her with her expensive race bike, which was *bent*, but fixable.

Cheryl was finally ready for physical therapy.

"Stan, the physical therapist, came to the house and helped me roll over onto my stomach, like doing a 'log roll.' He then started bending my knees. They would barely bend at first and it was very painful."

Most of us take walking for granted, and Cheryl had to learn how to do it all over again.

"Stan helped me learn to stand, which was very painful. At first, I could only stand for a few seconds because of the pain. I wondered if I would ever be able to stand for long. The blood would pool in my crushed left foot, causing incredible pain."

As a disciplined triathlete and hard worker, Cheryl was determined to get through the pain and learn to walk again.

*"After working on it day after day, I was finally able to stand for one minute...my son timed me. **We celebrated!"***

Cheryl's left leg was now one inch shorter than her right leg which required a "lift" in her left shoe.

"Over time, I learned to stand and walk with a walker, then with crutches, then one crutch, then a cane, then by myself."

Cheryl then began making trips to the hospital therapy building where she began exercising in water, coupled with some light swimming.

*"Swimming helped me with strength and endurance without causing me extra pain...but it seemed that my life was consumed with **'hard work, rest, and repeat.'"***

Several years later, Cheryl's right hip became so painful that she had to have it replaced.

"Doctor Blasingame did the hip surgery this time. He is an excellent surgeon. He also shortened my right leg to match my left leg...no more putting lifts in my left shoes!"

Cheryl found a way to compete in the Kalispell, Foy's Lake Triathlon not long after her hip replacement. She completed the ½-mile swim, 13-mile bike and 3.1-mile run, but one foot would continually "drop" as she ran, making running very difficult. (I also competed in that same triathlon and did not catch up with Cheryl until shortly before the finish line!)

After numerous tests and x-rays concerning her "dropping foot," she has finally decided to give up on ever running again, which was one of the joys in her life.

In February of 2019, Cheryl continues to have pains from that accident many years ago:

"A nerve was displaced in my left elbow that still gives me pain every time I bend that arm."

And...

"I must comb hair over a bare spot where a clump of my scalp was damaged."

Even today, over 28 years later, Cheryl continues to lose teeth from damaged nerves in her jaw. Cheryl says she has, "...spent thousands of dollars on the teeth."

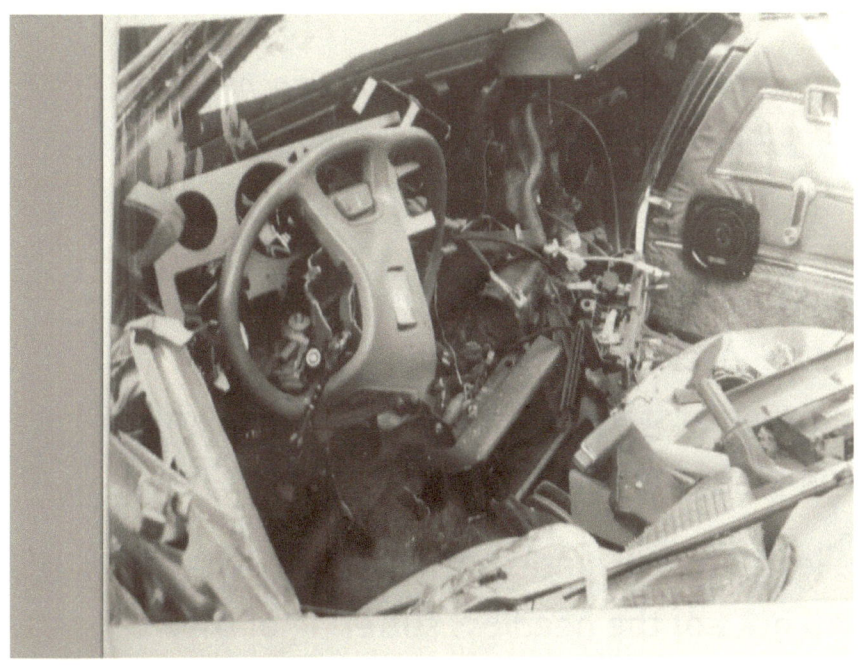

Amazingly, even though she now lives a life of "rebuilt roadkill," Cheryl does not harbor an angry attitude towards the woman who took her husband's life and who damaged her own body so badly.

"I suppose it was a good thing that it happened to us and not [other people] someone else."

This is one person's tragic story about survival after a senseless person drank alcohol, and in that drugged state, got behind the wheel of an automobile...not once, but many times.

The legislators in states such as Arizona have taken note of the needless suffering of their citizens and have taken steps to correct the problem with ignition/breathalyzer restrictions and severe penalties.

What are Montana legislators doing?

The Montana <u>Daily Inter Lake</u> newspaper reported on Saturday, January 19, 2019 that Montana State Senator Ed Buttrey recently submitted House Bill 35 to award Montana liquor licenses by an auction system, instead of the current lottery.

He estimates the auction system should generate between 2-$4 million more than the lotto system. Senator Buttrey admitted that he owns bars and casinos in the Flathead area and around Great Falls, but said the bill would not affect him.

I think we all should be asking the questions:

What is most important?

...dollar amounts in city and state coffers?

...or the lives and well-being of us citizens?

...and what are our legislators doing about it?

Sobriety checkpoints are a well-known means of stopping drunk drivers in their tracks, as reported by MADD, "Mothers Against Drunk Driving."[27]

Unfortunately, Montana is one of 12 states in the union that considers sobriety checkpoints unconstitutional.[28]

Does anyone besides me have a problem with this?

Why not mandatory breathalyzer/ignition locks with the first DUI?

Why not vehicle impounding with the first DUI?

Why not a lowered BAC to 0.05%?

Why not sobriety checkpoints like the majority of the country?

Why not longer stays in prison?

If prisons are full, why are the guilty not out picking up roadside litter?

I will leave it to the reader to decide who benefits from increased alcohol monies and weak Montana alcohol laws.

I doubt that it is Cheryl and Vernon Ward.

At the close of the interview, Cheryl's last words to me were:

"My life would have been so

different if not for a drunk driver."

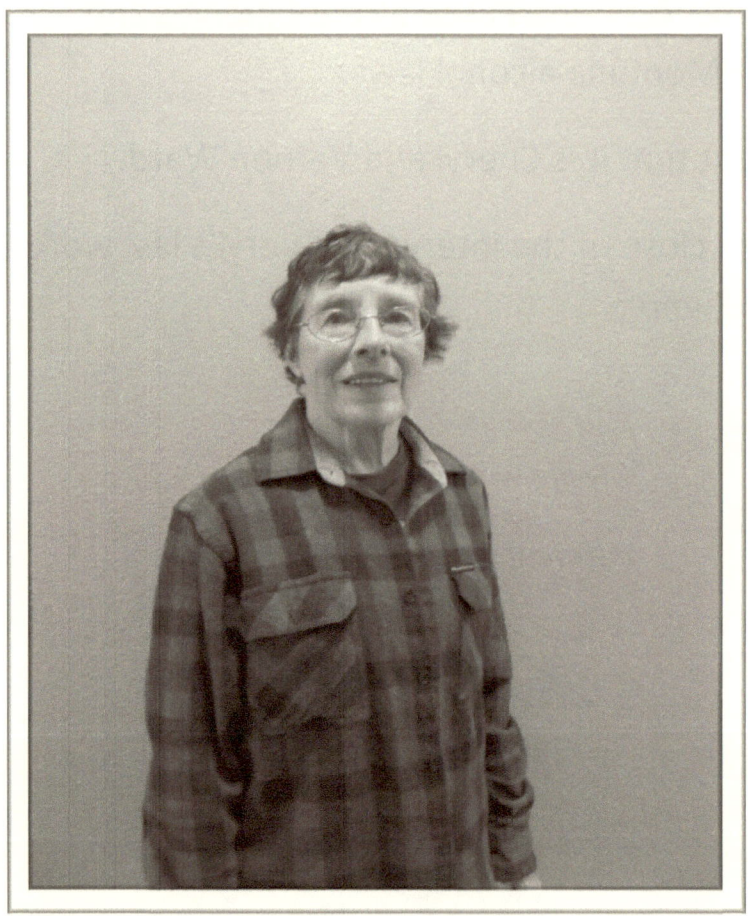

and...

"I miss Vern every day. We had plans."

Footnotes

1. www.healthdata.org/ Richard Horton/no-safe-level-of-alcohol, Aug. 23,2018 [Jan. 21, 2019]
2. www.labroots.com/ Brenda Kelley/ alcohol-unsafe-amount/ Aug. 28, 2018 [Jan. 21, 2019]
3. Ibid [Jan. 21, 2019]
4. https://pubs.niaa.nih.gov/ publications/Samir Zakhari, Ph.D., Overview: How is Alcohol Metabolized in the Body? [Jan. 21, 2019]
5. Montana Driver Manual, p. 71 [Jan. 21, 2019]
6. https://media.dojmt.gov/ substance use in Montana, pgs. 6-7, Sept., 2007 [Jan. 21, 2019]
7. Ibid, p. 23
8. https://mtstandard.com/ liquor-license-sale-database [Jan. 21, 2019]
9. https://pubs.niaaa.nih.gov/ publications/alcohol facts and stats/alcohol-related deaths [Jan. 21, 2019]
10. www.encyclopedia.com/ education/Advertising and the Alcohol Industry/Advertising Expenditures [Jan. 21, 2019]
11. www.newsadvance.com/ work_it_lynchburg/news/anheuser-busch/Anheuser-Busch Will Invest 2 Billion…[Jan. 22, 2019]

12. www.bustle.com/ articles/126692-this-elf-drinking-game...elf drinking game...buzzed with Buddy [Jan. 22, 2019]

13. www.verywellfamily.com/ Buddy T./par. 4/teens influenced/ Oct. 13, 2008 [Jan. 22, 2019]

14. www.vulture.com/ 2010/09/cougar_town_drinking, The Most Pro-Alcohol Show On TV, Willa Paskin, 9-30-10 [Jan. 22, 2019]

15. https://missoulian.com/ news/state-and-regional/legislature-is-rife..., Jayme Fraser, 7-2-17 [Jan. 22, 2019]

16. https://wallethub.com/ edu/dui-penalties-by-state/13549/#overall-rankings/Alina Comoreanu/8-10-17 [Jan. 22, 2019]

17. www.abc15.com/ money/Arizona-ranks-at-the-top..., Angie Koehle/8-12-16/ [Jan. 22, 2019]

18. www.wallethub.com/ edu/dui-penalties-by-state/overall rankings/Jayme Fraser, 7-2-17 [Jan 22, 2019]

19. https://helenair.com/ lifestyles/alcohol-fatality-rate-in-montana-is-the-worst-in-the/article, par. 4, Michael Jamison, 5-31-09 [Jan. 22, 2019]

20. https://helenair.com/ news/local/long-road-ahead-in-changing-states-dui-culture/article, Tristan Scott, 5-6-10 [Jan. 22, 2019]

21. www.mdt.mt.gov/ visionzero/docs/dui_penalties.pdf, 6-2017 [Jan. 22, 2019]

22. https://helenair.com/ news/local/long-road-ahead-in-changing-states-dui-culture [Jan. 22, 2019]

23. Ibid

24. www.intoxalock.com/ blog/post/Utah-to-implement…, 12-20-18, [Jan. 22, 2019]

25. www.zeroduideaths.org/ Montana DUI Task Force and Judges DUI Survey Analysis and Recommendations, [Jan. 22, 2019]

26. Used by permission of Cheryl Ward [Jan. 22, 2019]

27. www.madd.org/ sobriety checkpoints, 7-2018 [Jan. 22, 2019]

28. https://dui.laws.com/ checkpoint/ All You Need To Know About Checkpoints, par. 3, [Jan. 22, 2019]

29. www.cdc.gov/ features/costofdrinking/intex.html [Jan. 23, 2019]

30. www.futurity.org/ alcohol-light-drinking-risk-1882302, Jim Dryden-WUSTL [Jan. 25, 2019]

31. www.vice.com/ en_us/article/exm7y4/how-much-you-can-drink-before-it-can-kill-you-991, Mike Pearl, 12-11-14 [Jan. 25, 2019]

32. Ibid

33. www.alcohol.org.ng/ alcohol-its-effects/health-effects-alcohol-poisoning [Jan. 25, 2019

34. www.drinkamerican.US/who-owns-what-beers, [March 3, 2019]

35. https://money.cnn.com/2014/09/19/news/companies/pabst-oasis/index.html [March 3, 2019]

Kalispell Police Blotter

The following are actual alcohol-related events as posted in the Kalispell, Montana, Daily Inter Lake newspaper in 2018 and 2019.

Someone called 911 because they saw drunk people doing cartwheels.

A woman wearing a green bandanna was in a store drinking a beer and asking other customers at gas pumps for a ride to Polson. She was counseled about having an open container.

A store employee overheard two teen girls talking about drinking and doing drugs at a party.

An intoxicated pedestrian on Sixth Street was stumbling, cussing, not acting normal and yelling at cars.

A security company told officers a drunk man, described as "rail skinny" and carrying a green and black snowboard, was reportedly walking around and threatening to fight people.

A couch-crashing woman got drunk and punched her host four to six times in addition to throwing and breaking his vape pipe. The parties were separated and he reportedly did not wish to pursue charges, but had his mother picked up until she sobered up.

A drunk emergency room patient reportedly threatened to "go kill the people who beat him up," off Farm to Market Road.

A person reported what sounded to him like a drunken man who was lying face-down on a boat dock. The caller did not know if he was breathing and did not want to check. The man in question then got up and staggered away.

A man attempted to steal 2 beers from a Kalispell store, but an employee chased and caught the man as they wrestled and fought in the parking lot. The thief bit the employee and ran to his truck, but the employee pulled him back out of the truck and pinned him to the ground. Police officers responded and arrested the beer thief while paramedics responded to the bite victim.

A group of teens were busted for drinking and smoking marijuana at a party. The teens were detained and released to their parents.

A caller reported a drunk dad getting a haircut with his kids. An officer called the man's wife who drove them home. The wife was sober.

Two men were yelling at one another in a bar which turned into a wrestling match. One man's glasses were broken in the incident.

A stocky man with slicked-back hair slapped a woman at a Kalispell bar and then tried to fight four other men outside the bar.

A drunk pedestrian was reported stumbling in and out of Highway 35.

Two women between the ages of 18-20 were seen approaching men in a gas station parking lot off Highway 2, asking them if they wanted to buy alcohol.

A woman was seen drinking and smoking marijuana while driving a white Ford Taurus on Highway 2 with a child in the car. Officers were unable to locate the vehicle.

A caller on Highway 35 reported a man drinking and fighting with his wife. He said when his friend drinks that he gets belligerent.

A "very drunk" man reportedly left an establishment on Hodgson Road and was last seen swerving all over the road and speeding.

A reported verbal disturbance outside a local motel was defined by the parties involved as a, "simple drunken discussion."

A woman reported meeting a drunken man at a gas station. She knew he was drunk because he said he was drunk.

The man then sped off where officers chased him on the Highway 93 bypass.

The offender drove dangerously fast through the round-abouts.

Officers were able to stop and arrest the man.

A caller reported he was locked inside a bar that had closed for the night. He could not find his cell phone and was too drunk to drive home. He said an alarm was going off. The man was advised to sit still and not touch anything while someone came to let him out.

A family's park outing was cut short by a man wearing a red bandana and smelling of alcohol who kept trying to take their dog. The drunk man then filmed them with his phone.

Someone reported seeing a beer can fall out of a man's car in the parking lot of a grocery store. The man picked up the can and tossed into a shopping cart before stumbling into the store.

Twelve-year-olds were reportedly living in tents down by the river on an "older gentleman's" property, drinking and smoking.

A male driver was reported yelling, speeding and swerving while throwing beer cans from his SUV.

A drunk male was reported wandering around the Kalispell hospital campus. The caller was concerned because he said his friend always acts up when he is drunk. The man was eventually reunited with family who took him home.

A man was reported sitting in a truck drinking beer.

A very drunk young male was reportedly harassing people in a grocery store parking lot and trying to start fights. He then repeatedly tried breaking into unlocked cars. The male was reportedly falling-down-drunk who then started running towards a nearby fire hall. Police officers caught up with him and placed him under arrest.

A woman reported giving a transient a key to her storage shed so he could store his things. The transient was now drunk, screaming and causing a scene. Officers were warned the man could be hostile and very violent towards police.

A passerby reported a man threw a beer can out of a black truck while stopped at a light and proceeded to open another beer.

An employee at a bar on Highway 35 was trying to close up and wanted help in getting a homeless drunk out.

A shirtless man was seen hanging out the rear window of a moving silver sedan with a beer in hand making "hand gestures" to people. The sedan was reportedly being driven recklessly.

Some Kalispell kids grabbed a pair of 30-packs of beer and ran from the store. There was surveillance footage of the incident.

A drunk female was discovered passed out in her Hummer at a gas station. She was given a ride home.

A drunken woman with an open container would not leave a store.

A 17 to 19-year-old male with dark curly hair stole a six-pack of beer from a store on Highway 2 in Kalispell.

A woman who was slurring her words called from Seventh Street claiming someone keeps spreading rumors about her and she wants them to stop.

A woman tried to help a drunken man by picking him up and attempting to take him to multiple addresses. No one else wanted him and she eventually dropped him off at the police station.

A strong woman threw a dresser at a man that cut his face. Alcohol was suspected.

Dispatchers received a call and heard someone yelling, "My 33-year-old son is drunk and causing problems." At least two other couples could be heard arguing outside.

A driver who "seemed out of it," was suspected to be driving under the influence of alcohol, forgot his glasses and could not see.

A man reportedly under the influence of alcohol was "talking crazy stuff" about his girlfriend being in a jar and his dead parents in the street.

Someone said a couple who appeared to be under the influence of alcohol "could barely walk straight." The couple was spotted getting into a vehicle and driving westbound on Flathead Avenue.

Someone on Ninth Street requested officers do a walk-through after denying service to a man with missing teeth who was reportedly talking to himself after a beer and shot of whiskey.

A woman on Lakeshore Drive requested extra patrols around her apartment after finding alcohol cans at the bottom of her stairs.

A Kalispell woman took out a restraining order against a building contractor she had fired earlier in the day after he returned to the work site, drunk and disorderly.

An inebriated woman slurring her words called from Seventh Street to report someone keeps spreading rumors about her and she wants them to stop.

A woman called to report her alcoholic, incoherently-wasted son was not supposed to be at her house.

A Good Samaritan picked up a drunken male at a bar and attempted to give him a ride to a home. However, no one was home and he wanted to know what to do with the drunk in his car.

A drunk male driver was seen speeding, swerving, yelling, cussing and throwing beer cans from his SUV.

A woman was worried that her sixty-three-year-old friend might freeze outside after drinking a couple pints of vodka and refusing to come inside.

A man under the influence of alcohol fell and suffered a cut on his head. He claimed his son or niece caused him to fall. He then changed his story and said his brother did it. He finally admitted that he did not know what happened, but thought someone had hit him on the back of the head, causing him to fall. He refused medical help.

A middle-aged man wearing sunglasses and cowboy hat was reported as "obviously drunk" while seated behind the wheel of his pickup truck.

A man called 911 claiming he had been robbed and knocked out. He thought he had been unconscious for about thirty minutes after waking up in a snow drift a couple of blocks from his home with cash and credit cards missing. The man was covered in blood with a large bump on his head, but refused medical help.

A drunk woman in skinny jeans was reported stumbling along a sidewalk. She fell into a snow bank and later onto the ground. Her boyfriend eventually showed up to get her.

A driver on Highway 82 reported another driver who was parked and slumped over his steering wheel. That driver then drove down the middle of the road. The vehicle stopped at Mc Caffery Road where the driver vomited out a window. He then attempted to turn around, which was when the caller stopped following him.

A drunk woman was reported standing by the pumps at a gas station on Highway 2 for over an hour.

A driver reported almost running over a man lying in the middle of the road. The man was described as "tall and thin." The man then got up and staggered down the road.

A drunk caller on Shady Lane reported his belief that deputies were trying to kill him.

A drunk woman would not leave a Kalispell store.

A female bartender said her co-workers, who were drinking, were accusing her of not doing her job because she got a little behind while serving a large group.

A drunk and partially-clad woman was reported walking down the middle of Highway 93. She was described as having blonde hair, wearing a white jacket, but no pants. She had a bicycle with her but left it when officers took her to the hospital.

A thirty-three-year-old man called 911 to report that he had been drinking alcohol heavily for several days, was sick and thought he might have alcohol poisoning. He said he had been shaking and vomiting. It was learned that he was on probation for criminal endangerment and possession of dangerous drugs as well as possessing various types of guns.

A drunk, homeless woman reported that her drunk and homeless fiancé hit her while they were trying to go to sleep. She said he then ran off into the woods. The woman was advised to not sleep under the bridge.

A woman reported her drunk boyfriend had slapped her in the face which made her bleed. She added that the boyfriend was now standing in the front yard waiting for deputies to come and take him to jail.

A mom brought her sixteen-year-old daughter to the police station for a breathalyzer test because she thought she had been drinking alcohol.

A man rolled his vehicle somewhere between Kalispell and Missoula in the night but managed to get a ride to the hospital in Kalispell. After waking from surgery, he had no idea where the accident had taken place. Alcohol was suspected.

A caller on Second Street was concerned about a man who had fallen while attempting to cross the street. The caller thought the man was drunk. He said it took the staggering man over two minutes to cross the street. Officers arrived, but the man said he did not need any help.

A drunk male wearing an orange hat and camo jacket was reported for stealing $2-3 worth of yogurt from a store. An officer detained the man but the store refused to press charges.

Someone reported a store cashier had been drinking alcohol while on her lunch break. She refused to leave the store, but finally did so after officers were called and made her leave.

A woman called 911 for help in getting her phone out of emergency mode. She sounded drunk to dispatch after slurring her words and failing to properly repeat the phrase, "She sells sea shells."

A drunk and very agitated man came to the police station to complain about being tossed out of a local bar because he asked for a black trash bag.

A man reported his wife for being, "drunk and dramatic."

A drunk male wearing camouflage clothing was reportedly asleep in the middle of a road with his arm around a bag of groceries.

A man was cited for public drunkenness after someone reported him for urinating along the side of a road. He was also trying to ride a bicycle but kept falling off.

A red-haired woman was reported for throwing glasses and breaking things at a bar. She was last seen walking down the road wearing a short red skirt and jeans jacket.

An extremely drunk twenty-three-year-old male was found in the park after hours. He was so drunk that he did not know where he lived and urinated in the back of the patrol car.

A man was reported as "flailing" on the ground. A deputy determined the man was just drunk.

A man known to deputies as,
"chronically intoxicated," called to
report 20 people on Managhan Lane
with machinery and guns. The man
insisted on knowing what was going
on. Officers determined nothing
unusual was taking place.

A bouncer in a bar reported the drunk
he had just kicked out of the
establishment was now urinating on
the side of the building.

A bartender reported two men fighting in front of the bar. An officer told the men to move along. The men returned later and the bartender had to kick them out again.

An inebriated man called and asked for a welfare check on himself as to why he was slurring his words.

An employee at a fast food store checked on a drunk found asleep in the snow. She roused him and asked if he needed help. The man refused help, saying he was okay.

A man told dispatch that he had a small emergency that could only be shared with a male officer. A deputy contacted the man who said he desperately needed a six-pack of beer and a carton of Swisher Sweets cigars.

The man was informed that law enforcement could not fulfill his request.

A man called 911 because he had been drinking in a bar and saw the man who assaulted his brother two weeks ago. He wanted officers to check the man out. Deputies arrived and determined it was not him.

Someone reported trying to say "hi" to a stranger in a parking lot. The man replied with, "You're lucky you are not dead." Officers said the stranger had been removed from the premises the previous day for attempting to steal beer.

A man was sure he had his phone when entering a bar and now cannot find it.

A woman reported that when she and her boyfriend were drinking in a bar, they overheard another man talking about how he had killed a man the day before.

A caller was upset at a female bartender when she would not give him "a gosh-darn drink."

Someone was trying to help an alcoholic friend by letting him stay the night, but the *alky* became rude and unruly. The caller wanted deputies to come and get him.

A woman reported her boyfriend suffered a broken jaw in a fight behind a bar where he had been drinking, and she was trying to sort things out since he could not talk.

A janitor let a man with a beard and large backpack into a bar through the back door and he slipped out without paying for his beer and beer nuts.

Someone reported a man passed out at a bar after a night of heavy drinking. When officers could not rouse the man, they called paramedics who took him to the hospital where it was learned he had suffered a stroke.

Someone reported a drunk male stumbling and falling down on Pheasant Run.

A drunk man was reported falling down with a bottle of wine and trying to kiss passengers outside the train station.

Someone reported three men and two women in a bar brawl.

A man assaulted the DJ at a bar and tried to fight two other people inside. Two women also fought at the bar. One man had a head injury, but no one wanted to press charges.

A woman was taken into custody for drunken driving after driving her car into a ditch along Darlington Street. The woman almost fell out of her vehicle when someone checked on her.

An officer gave a woman a ride who he found wandering along Second Avenue with a bottle of wine in hand. The woman needed help getting up a flight of stairs.

A man was seen stumbling down Glenwood Drive wearing a stocking cap, carrying a backpack and toting a plastic bag. He was also observed urinating in the street.

A woman on Flathead Avenue called to see if she had left her phone in a jail cell. She said she and her husband had spent the night there after drinking too much the previous night and doing something that caused them to end up in a holding cell.

A woman was removed from a house on Park Avenue after drinking three bottles of wine and kicking someone.

After a man was reported running around the neighborhood in his pajamas, he told officers he was pretty sure he was drunk because he could not remember his name.

A drunk male was reported sleeping in the middle of the intersection at Third Street and Sixth Avenue.

Someone reported finding a very drunk woman sleeping on the back seat of their car parked on Central Avenue. When they told her to get out, she lay down on the pavement in the parking lot.

Officers responded to two calls about injured males after a fight at a bar on Central Avenue.

After a night of drinking, a woman reported finding yellow "evidence tape" on one of her windows. She was calling to find out what had happened the previous night.

A bartender on First Avenue reported someone tried paying him with a counterfeit $100 bill.

A caller reported the car in front of him weaving all over the road. He followed it to a bar where a woman stumbled out and went into the bar. An officer arrived, went inside and found the female who had been driving the car and arrested her for DUI.

A driver reported a man stumbling in and out of Central Avenue. Officers found the man leaning against a building who said he thought he could find his way home on his own.

A woman called to report a man with her who had been in a violent rage all day. She handed her phone to the man who said he just wanted to go to sleep. The woman said the man had kicked her, and she then hung up.

Dispatch called back, but learned that no one had actually been kicked in the shin during the incident.

The same woman called one hour later and asked the dispatcher to pray for her because her friend was drinking again.

The woman called once again forty-five minutes later, asking for an ambulance. She thought that might scare him.

EMT's arrived and cleared the man medically.

The woman called a short time later, crying, saying she could not drive and wondered if she should call a cab for the man.

An officer tried to close the call but she hung up. She called once again a short time later, very distraught, asking to speak with an officer.

The woman hung up, but called right back again asking for an officer and wondered if there might be a program in town where the drunk man might work with children.

The woman hung up, but called again to thank dispatchers.

In her final call, the woman invited all the deputies and dispatchers over to her place for an early Thanksgiving dinner.

The woman called dispatch a total of ten times in a twelve-hour period.

The woman's dinner invitation was politely declined.

About the author

In the year 2019, Joe Apple is a 10-year resident of Montana, married for 47 years to the same woman and father of 2 children from that union.

Joe is a retired instructor for the California Bureau of Automobile Repair, specializing in computer diagnostics. He also served as editor and proofreader for technical manuals produced for use throughout the state of California.

Joe earned a 4-year BA art degree from Point Loma Nazarene University, class of 2003, in San Diego, California.

Joe was a California, state-certified Emergency Medical Technician and Certified Nurse Assistant.

Joe has volunteered in hospital emergency rooms for 1,700 hours over the course of 16 years in the states of California and Montana.

Joe may be contacted at applecor3@gmail.com.